Live Comfortably with IRRITABLE BOWEL SYNROME

A Doctor's Practical Guide to Understanding & Managing IBS

Dr Prabhat Das

MD, PhD, FACP

Better Health with Dr Das Series

Hardcover ISBN: 978-1-971672-30-4

Paperback ISBN: 978-1-971672-29-8

eBook ISBN: 978-1-971672-28-1

Printed in the United States of America

Disclaimer

This book is intended solely for educational and informational purposes. It is not meant to replace personal medical advice, diagnosis, or treatment.

Although I am a licensed physician, reading this book does not establish a doctor-patient relationship. Each individual's health condition, medical history, and risk factors are unique. Any medical decision should be made in partnership with your own healthcare professional who understands your specific situation.

Medical science is continually advancing. New research and updated guidelines may lead to changes in recommendations over time.

About the Author

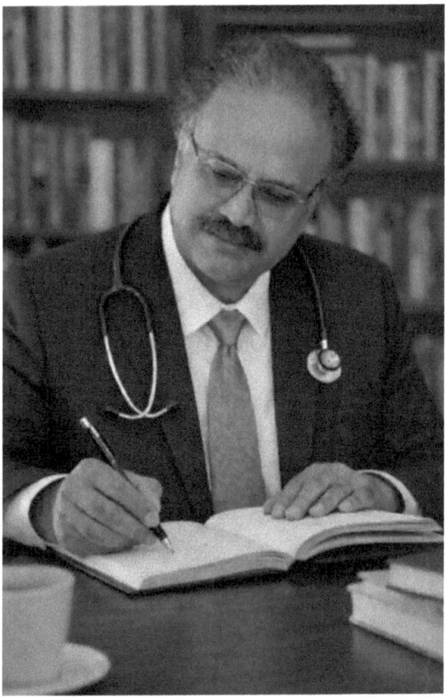

I am Dr Prabhat Das, MD, PhD, FACP. My journey in medicine began in India and, over the past thirty-five years, has continued in the United States, where I have had the privilege of caring for patients across a wide range of medical settings. I am trained in Internal Medicine, Pulmonary Diseases, and Critical Care. For me, medicine has never been just a profession. It has been a lifelong commitment shaped by learning, service, and a deep respect for the trust patients place in their physician.

Over the years, I have had the honor of caring for patients in many different situations. I have seen individuals in my office for routine concerns, treated urgent conditions in busy emergency rooms, managed serious illnesses in the hospital, and cared for critically ill patients in intensive care units. Each setting has taught me something valuable. Each patient has added to my understanding of what it truly means to care for another human being.

But one lesson has stood above all others. Medicine is not only about tests, diagnoses, or treatments. It is about people. It is about listening carefully, understanding fears that are often left unspoken, and guiding patients through uncertainty with clarity and compassion. Again and again, I have seen that what people want most is simple, trustworthy information. They want to understand what is happening in their bodies. They want to feel confident about the decisions they are making for their health and for their families.

These experiences have deeply shaped how I think about health, illness, prevention, and the human side of healing.

That is the reason behind the '**Better Health with Dr Das Series'**. Through these books, I hope to reach individuals I may never meet in person but who are searching for clear and reliable guidance. In today's world, health information is everywhere, yet much of it is confusing, overwhelming, and sometimes misleading. My goal is to cut through that noise and present important medical topics in a way that is simple, practical, and reassuring.

Every page of this series is guided by two foundations: reliable scientific knowledge and decades of real-world clinical experience. I want you, the reader, to feel informed, confident, and empowered. Not overwhelmed. Not confused. But clear about what you can do, step by step, to improve your health.

If even one reader feels less anxious, more informed, or better prepared to take control of their health after reading these books, then this work has served its purpose.

Helping people live healthier, longer, more confident and better-informed lives remains one of the greatest privileges of my life.

TABLE OF CONTENTS:

INTRODUCTION

Understanding Your Gut, Regaining Your Life

Over the years, I have met countless patients who walked into my office with a very similar story.

They were not severely ill. Their tests were often normal. Many had already seen other doctors. Yet, something in their daily life was clearly not right.

They would describe a pattern that had slowly taken hold of their routine.

A discomfort in the abdomen that came and went without warning. A feeling of fullness or bloating that made even simple meals uncomfortable. Sudden urgency that made them anxious about stepping out of the house. Or days of constipation that left them feeling heavy, frustrated, and incomplete.

And almost always, at some point in the conversation, they would say something like this:

"Doctor, everything looks normal, but I do not feel normal."

That one sentence, simple yet deeply meaningful, captures the essence of irritable bowel syndrome, or IBS.

IBS is one of the most common conditions affecting the digestive system. Yet, it is also one of the most misunderstood. Many patients live with symptoms for years without a clear explanation. Some are told not to worry. Others are told it is just stress.

Many are left in a state of confusion, trying different diets, avoiding foods, and constantly worrying about what might trigger their symptoms next.

Over time, this uncertainty begins to affect more than just the body.

It affects confidence.

Patients begin to plan their day around access to a restroom. They hesitate to travel. They avoid social gatherings. Some even begin to fear food itself.

This is where the real burden of IBS lies.

Not in the intestine alone, but in how it quietly interferes with daily life.

That is why I decided to write this book.

My goal is not to overwhelm you with medical terminology or complicated theories. Instead, I want to sit with you, almost like a quiet conversation, and explain IBS in a way that is clear, practical, and meaningful.

When you understand what is happening inside your body, something important begins to change.

Fear starts to fade.

When fear fades, you begin to observe instead of react. You begin to notice patterns. You make calmer, more informed decisions. And slowly, you begin to regain control over your body and your life.

In this book, we will walk step by step.

We will begin by understanding what IBS really is and, just as importantly, what it is not. We will explore why it develops, how the gut and brain interact, and why symptoms can feel so real even when tests are normal.

We will then move into the practical aspects that matter most in daily life.

You will learn how food affects your symptoms, not in a rigid or restrictive way, but in a balanced and thoughtful manner. We will discuss lifestyle habits, sleep, and physical activity. We will explore the role of stress, not as a cause to blame, but as a factor to understand and manage.

We will also discuss medications in a clear and sensible way, so that you can use them wisely when needed. And importantly, we will talk about real-life situations such as work, travel, and social life, because that is where IBS truly affects you.

There is one message I want to make very clear from the beginning.

IBS is real, but it is not dangerous.

It does not damage your intestine. It does not lead to cancer. But it can affect your comfort and quality of life if it is not understood properly.

The good news is this.

With the right knowledge and a steady, patient approach, IBS can be managed very effectively. Most patients improve significantly. Many return to a comfortable and confident daily life.

You do not need to rush through this book.

Read it slowly. Reflect on your own experience. Make small, practical changes.

Improvement in IBS does not come from sudden, dramatic changes.

It comes from steady understanding and consistent effort.

Think of this book as a guide, but also as a companion.

We will move forward step by step.

CHAPTER 1: What Is IBS

A Simple Beginning

Let us begin with a clear and honest understanding.

Irritable bowel syndrome, or IBS, is a condition in which the digestive system does not function in a smooth and predictable way, even though it appears normal on routine medical tests.

There are no ulcers. No tumors. No visible damage.

Yet, the symptoms are very real.

This often confuses patients.

"How can everything be normal when I feel so uncomfortable?"

The answer lies in understanding the difference between **structure and function**.

Function vs Structure: The Key Concept

In many diseases, we see a structural problem.

For example, an ulcer in the stomach or inflammation in the intestine. These can be seen on tests.

IBS is different.

In IBS, the structure of the intestine is normal, but the way it works is altered.

Think of it like a well-built car with no visible damage, but the engine is not running smoothly.

Everything looks fine, but the performance is not right.

That is IBS.

What Happens Inside the Gut

There are two main changes that occur in IBS.

First, the movement of the intestine becomes irregular.

The bowel may move too quickly, leading to loose stools or diarrhea. Or it may move too slowly, leading to constipation. In many people, it alternates between the two.

Second, the intestine becomes more sensitive.

Normal processes like digestion, movement of food, or even small amounts of gas may cause discomfort or pain.

What most people would not even notice can feel quite intense in someone with IBS.

This increased sensitivity is a key feature.

Why the Symptoms Feel So Real

Many patients struggle with this idea.

"If nothing is damaged, why does it hurt?"

This is an important question.

The answer lies in the nerves of the intestine.

In IBS, these nerves become more responsive. They send stronger signals to the brain.

At the same time, the brain becomes more aware of these signals.

This leads to a situation where normal activity inside the gut feels uncomfortable or even painful.

So the pain is not imagined.

It is very real.

A Common but Often Hidden Condition

IBS is extremely common.

A large number of people experience symptoms at some point in their lives, but many never talk about it.

Some feel embarrassed to discuss bowel habits. Others are told that nothing serious is wrong and are left without a clear explanation.

As a result, many people live with IBS quietly, adjusting their lives without truly understanding what is happening.

If you are one of them, it is important to know this.

You are not alone.

IBS Is Not a Dangerous Disease

Let me reassure you clearly.

IBS does not cause cancer. It does not damage your intestine. It does not lead to serious disease.

This is very important.

However, even though it is not dangerous, it can affect your quality of life.

And that is why it deserves attention.

How IBS Affects Daily Life

IBS is not just about bowel movement.

It affects how you live your day.

You may think twice before going out. You may worry about food. You may feel uncomfortable during meetings or travel.

Over time, this can affect your confidence.

Some patients begin to plan their entire day around their symptoms.

This is where IBS becomes more than just a digestive issue.

It becomes a lifestyle issue.

IBS Is Different in Every Person

No two patients with IBS are exactly the same.

Some have mostly constipation. Others have diarrhea. Some have both.

Some have mild symptoms. Others have more persistent discomfort.

This variation is normal.

It also means that treatment must be personalized.

What works for one person may not work for another.

A Condition You Can Understand and Manage

Here is the most important message from this chapter.

IBS is not something mysterious.

It can be understood.

And once it is understood, it can be managed.

You may not be able to control every symptom completely.

But you can reduce their frequency, intensity, and impact on your life.

And that makes a big difference.

What is IBS?

A Functional Disorder

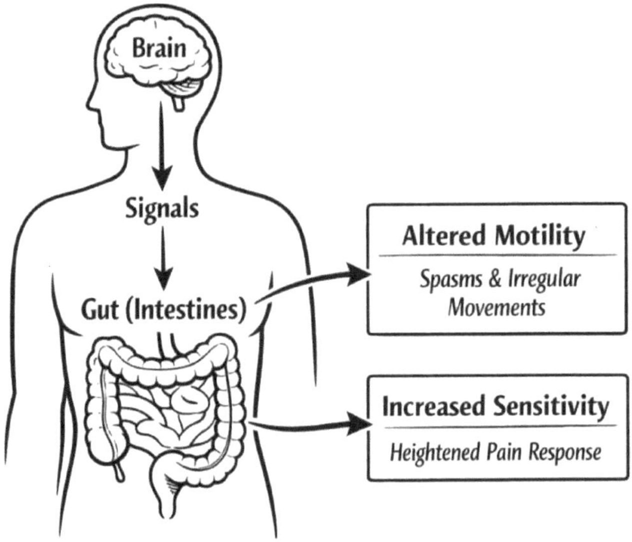

Normal Tests—But Real Symptoms.

Chapter Summary

- IBS is a disorder of function, not structure
- The intestine looks normal but does not work smoothly
- Movement of the bowel becomes irregular
- The gut becomes more sensitive
- Symptoms are real even when tests are normal
- IBS is common but often misunderstood
- It is not dangerous but can affect daily life
- Each person's experience is different

Action Plan

- Begin to understand your symptoms without fear
- Remind yourself that IBS is real but not dangerous
- Start observing patterns in your digestion
- Avoid jumping to conclusions based on one bad day
- Prepare yourself to learn more in the next chapters

Transition to the Next Chapter

Now that you understand what IBS is, the next question naturally arises. Why does it happen?

What causes the gut to behave this way, and why does stress seem to affect it so much?

In the next chapter, we will explore this in depth.

CHAPTER 2: How IBS Develops

A Conversation You Cannot See, But Always Feel

Let me begin with a simple idea.

Your gut and your brain are constantly talking to each other.

This is not a theory. It is a well-established biological system involving nerves, hormones, and chemical signals. This communication happens all the time, quietly in the background, without your awareness.

But sometimes, you do notice it.

Before an important meeting, you may feel a flutter in your stomach. During a stressful day, your digestion may feel unsettled. On a relaxed day, your body may feel light and comfortable.

These are everyday examples of what we call the **gut–brain connection**.

In IBS, this connection becomes more sensitive, more reactive, and less balanced.

When the System Becomes Overactive

In a healthy person, communication between the gut and brain is smooth and well-regulated.

In IBS, this communication becomes exaggerated.

Small signals from the gut are amplified when they reach the brain. At the same time, signals from the brain can trigger stronger responses in the gut.

This creates a loop.

A minor change in digestion leads to a stronger signal to the brain. The brain reacts, which further disturbs the gut. Over time, this loop contributes to ongoing symptoms.

Understanding this loop is one of the most important steps in managing IBS.

Because what you understand, you can begin to control.

The Role of Gut Movement

The intestine is not a passive organ. It is constantly moving in a coordinated rhythm to push food forward.

In IBS, this rhythm becomes irregular.

Sometimes the bowel moves too quickly. Food passes through faster than normal, leading to loose stools or diarrhea.

At other times, movement slows down. This leads to constipation, with hard stools that are difficult to pass.

In many patients, these patterns alternate.

This is why IBS often feels unpredictable.

Increased Sensitivity: The Real Reason for Pain

One of the defining features of IBS is increased sensitivity of the gut.

In simple terms, the intestine reacts more strongly to normal activity.

A small amount of gas, which most people would not notice, may cause discomfort or even pain.

Normal stretching of the bowel during digestion may feel uncomfortable.

This is not because something is damaged.

It is because the nerves in the intestine are more responsive.

Think of it as turning up the volume on a speaker. Even a soft sound becomes loud.

The Role of Stress and Emotions

Stress plays a major role in IBS, but it is important to understand it correctly.

Stress does not mean the problem is "in your head."

It means your body is responding to signals from your brain.

When you are stressed, your body releases hormones such as cortisol and adrenaline. These affect the digestive system.

The bowel may speed up or slow down. Sensitivity increases. Pain feels stronger.

This is why many patients notice that their symptoms worsen during stressful periods.

There is also a cycle that develops.

Symptoms create worry. Worry increases stress. Stress worsens symptoms.

Breaking this cycle is a key part of treatment.

The Gut Microbiome: Your Inner Environment

Inside your intestine lives a large number of bacteria.

This is known as the **gut microbiome**.

These bacteria are not harmful. In fact, many of them are beneficial. They help in digestion, support the immune system, and even influence mood.

In IBS, this balance may be disturbed.

This can happen after an infection, after antibiotic use, or sometimes without a clear reason.

When the balance changes, it can affect gas production, digestion, and sensitivity.

Research in this area is growing, and it is becoming an important part of our understanding of IBS.

IBS After Infection

Some patients clearly remember when their symptoms began.

They had an episode of food poisoning or a stomach infection. The infection improved, but their digestion never returned to normal.

This is called **post-infectious IBS**.

In such cases, the intestine remains sensitive even after the infection is gone.

This explains why symptoms can persist long after the original illness.

Low-Level Irritation

In IBS, there is no major inflammation like in serious bowel diseases.

However, in some patients, there may be a mild, low-level irritation in the intestine.

This is not enough to cause damage, but it can increase sensitivity and alter function.

It is another piece of the puzzle.

The Role of Diet and Lifestyle

Diet and lifestyle do not cause IBS by themselves, but they influence how it behaves.

Certain foods can increase gas production. Irregular eating habits can disturb bowel rhythm. Poor sleep and lack of physical activity can worsen symptoms.

These factors do not create IBS, but they can trigger or aggravate it.

Etiologies of IBS

Common Contributing Factors

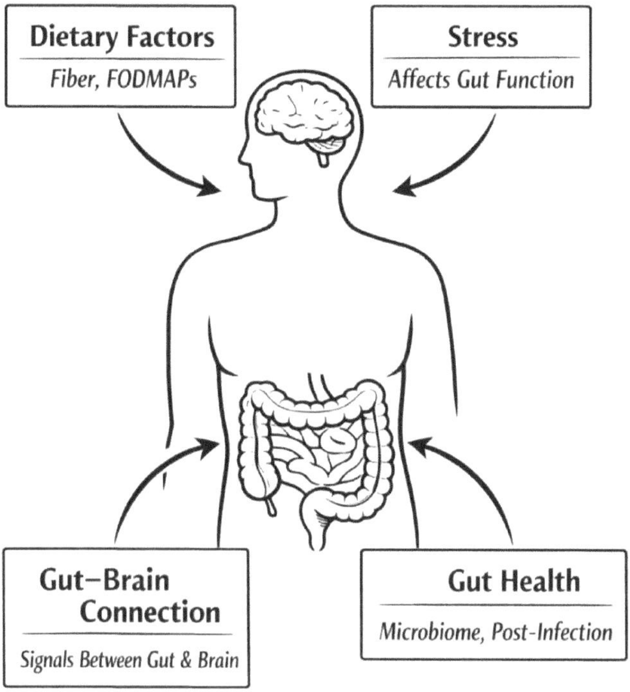

Multiple Factors Influence IBS

Why IBS Is Different in Each Person

IBS does not have a single cause.

It develops from a combination of factors:

- Sensitive gut–brain communication
- Irregular bowel movement
- Increased nerve sensitivity
- Changes in gut bacteria
- Effects of stress
- Lifestyle and dietary influences

Each person has a different combination of these factors.

That is why IBS looks different in different people.

Chapter Summary

- The gut and brain communicate constantly
- In IBS, this communication becomes exaggerated
- Bowel movement becomes irregular
- The gut becomes more sensitive
- Stress influences symptoms but is not the only cause
- The gut microbiome plays an important role
- IBS can develop after infections
- Multiple factors combine to produce symptoms

Action Plan

- Begin observing how stress affects your digestion

- Continue your symptom diary
- Note any past infections or antibiotic use
- Pay attention to lifestyle patterns
- Start viewing IBS as a whole-body condition

Transition to the Next Chapter

Now that you understand how IBS develops, the next step is to recognize its different patterns.

IBS does not present the same way in everyone.

In the next chapter, we will explore these patterns in detail and help you identify your own type.

CHAPTER 3: Types of IBS

Why Understanding Your Type Matters

By now, you understand what IBS is and how it develops.

The next step is very practical.

You need to understand your **pattern**.

IBS does not present the same way in everyone. Two patients may both have IBS, but their symptoms and daily challenges can be very different.

Recognizing your type helps in three important ways.

It reduces confusion.
It guides treatment decisions.
And it gives you a sense of control.

When you know your pattern, you stop guessing and start managing.

The Three Main Types of IBS

IBS is generally divided into three main types based on bowel habits:

- IBS with constipation
- IBS with diarrhea
- Mixed IBS

Let us look at each of these in a simple and practical way.

IBS with Constipation

In this type, constipation is the main issue.

Bowel movements may be infrequent. Stools are often hard, dry, and difficult to pass. You may need to strain, and even after passing stool, you may feel that the bowel has not emptied completely.

Bloating is often a major concern. Many patients describe a heavy, tight feeling in the abdomen, especially as the day progresses.

Abdominal discomfort or pain is common. It may improve slightly after a bowel movement, but not always completely.

This pattern can be frustrating because relief often feels incomplete.

IBS with Diarrhea

In this type, the bowel moves too quickly.

You may have frequent loose stools, sometimes several times a day. There is often urgency, a sudden need to pass stool, which can create anxiety, especially when you are outside.

Abdominal cramping is common and may come on suddenly. Passing stool often brings relief, but symptoms may return later.

One useful observation is that IBS symptoms usually occur during the day and rarely wake you from sleep.

This pattern can interfere with daily activities because of its unpredictability.

Mixed IBS

In mixed IBS, constipation and diarrhea both occur.

You may have a few days of constipation followed by days of loose stools. Sometimes the change happens quickly, making it difficult to predict.

This pattern can feel confusing.

Treatments that help at one time may not help at another.

Understanding that this is a recognized pattern helps reduce frustration.

Management requires flexibility and patience.

IBS Without a Clear Pattern

Not everyone fits neatly into one category.

Some patients have symptoms that vary in a way that does not follow a clear pattern.

This is still IBS.

The important thing is not the label, but understanding your own body.

Why Your Pattern May Change Over Time

IBS is not a fixed condition.

Your pattern may change.

A person with constipation may later develop diarrhea. Someone with diarrhea may occasionally experience constipation.

These changes can be influenced by:

- Diet
- Stress
- Medications
- Travel
- Infections
- Changes in routine

This does not mean that the disease is worsening.

It reflects the flexible nature of IBS.

Recognizing Your Own Pattern

You do not need complicated tests to understand your type.

Simple observation is enough.

Pay attention to:

- How often you pass stool
- The consistency of stool

- Whether you feel urgency or difficulty
- Whether you feel complete relief after a bowel movement

Your symptom diary will help you see patterns over time.

A Practical Tool: Stool Consistency

One useful way to understand your bowel pattern is to observe stool consistency.

You may notice:

- Hard, pellet-like stools → constipation pattern
- Soft or loose stools → diarrhea pattern
- Alternating → mixed pattern

This simple observation can guide your approach to diet and treatment.

Avoid Overanalyzing

While it is helpful to understand your pattern, it is equally important not to overanalyze every change.

IBS naturally fluctuates.

Instead of reacting to every variation, focus on overall trends.

A calm and balanced approach helps reduce anxiety and improves long-term control.

Types of IBS

Common Subtypes

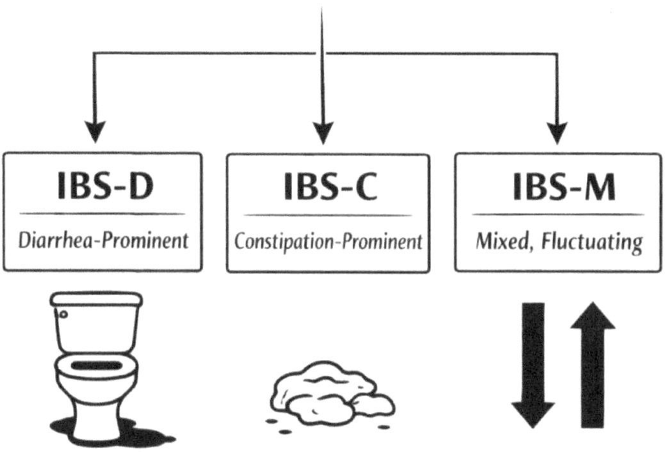

Different Patterns, Influence IBS

A Key Message

Understanding your type is not about labeling yourself.

It is about guiding your management.

Once you recognize your pattern, you can take more targeted and effective steps.

This is where control begins.

Chapter Summary

- IBS presents in different patterns based on bowel habits
- The three main types are constipation, diarrhea, and mixed
- Some patients do not fit neatly into one category
- Symptoms may change over time
- Simple observation helps identify your pattern
- Stool consistency is a useful guide
- Avoid overanalyzing daily changes
- Understanding your type helps guide treatment

Action Plan

- Continue your symptom diary
- Observe stool frequency and consistency
- Identify your predominant pattern over 2 to 3 weeks
- Note any changes related to diet, stress, or routine
- Focus on overall trends rather than daily variations

CHAPTER 4: Symptoms of IBS

Looking Beyond the Obvious

When most people think of IBS, they think only of constipation or diarrhea.

But in real life, IBS is much more than a change in bowel movement.

It is a collection of symptoms that can affect how you feel throughout the day, physically and emotionally. Some symptoms are obvious. Others are subtle but equally important.

Understanding the full picture helps you stay calm and in control.

When you recognize a symptom as part of IBS, it becomes less frightening and more manageable.

Abdominal Pain and Discomfort

Pain is one of the most common and important symptoms of IBS.

It is usually felt in the lower abdomen, but it can occur anywhere across the belly. The sensation may vary. Some patients describe it as cramping. Others describe it as a dull ache, pressure, or discomfort.

A key feature of IBS pain is its relationship to bowel movement.

The pain often improves after passing stool.

This is an important clue that helps distinguish IBS from other conditions.

Pain may increase after meals or during periods of stress. It usually comes and goes rather than remaining constant.

Even though tests are normal, the discomfort can be quite distressing.

Bloating: A Common and Disturbing Symptom

Bloating is one of the most frequently reported symptoms.

Patients often describe a feeling of fullness, tightness, or heaviness in the abdomen. Some feel that their abdomen becomes visibly swollen, especially as the day progresses.

Others may not see a visible change but still feel uncomfortable pressure inside.

This symptom is often worse after meals and toward the evening.

Bloating can affect not only comfort but also confidence.

Gas and Abdominal Distension

Closely related to bloating is the sensation of gas.

You may feel excessive gas, frequent passage of gas, or a sense of trapped gas.

In IBS, even normal amounts of gas can feel uncomfortable because of increased sensitivity.

Diet and gut bacteria both play a role in this symptom.

Changes in Bowel Habits

This is one of the defining features of IBS.

Some patients experience frequent loose stools or diarrhea. Others experience constipation, with hard stools and difficulty passing them.

Many experience both patterns at different times.

The bowel pattern may not remain consistent.

This variability is a hallmark of IBS.

Urgency and Loss of Control

Urgency is a sudden, strong need to pass stool. It can be difficult to delay and may create anxiety, especially in public settings.

Some patients feel the need to locate restrooms wherever they go.

This symptom can significantly affect daily life.

Symptoms of IBS

Common Symptoms

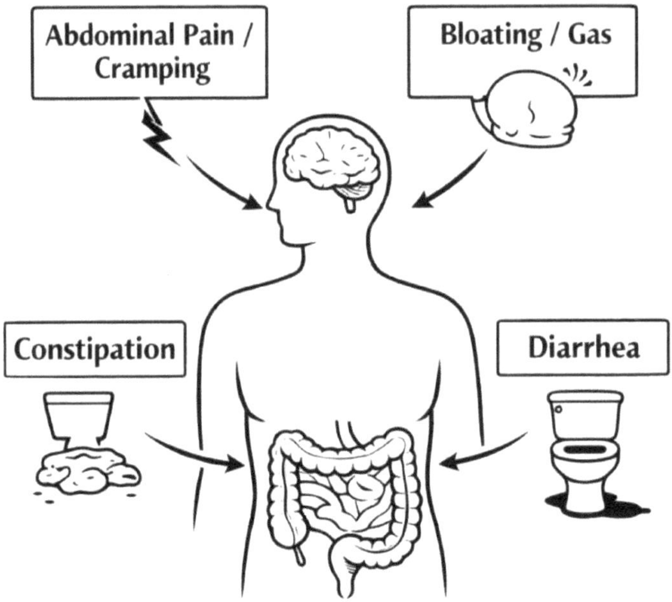

Symptoms Vary, But These Are Common

Incomplete Evacuation

Another common symptom is the feeling that the bowel has not emptied completely.

Even after passing stool, there may be a sense of fullness or the need to go again.

This can lead to repeated attempts and ongoing discomfort.

Mucus in Stool

Some patients notice mucus in their stool.

This may appear as a clear or whitish coating.

In IBS, this is usually harmless.

The intestine naturally produces mucus, and in IBS it may be more noticeable.

However, it is important to remember that blood in the stool is not a feature of IBS and should always be evaluated.

Fatigue and Low Energy

IBS does not only affect the gut.

Many patients report feeling tired or low in energy.

This may be due to poor sleep, ongoing discomfort, or the mental effort of managing symptoms.

Fatigue can affect concentration, work performance, and overall quality of life.

Sleep Disturbance

IBS symptoms usually do not wake you from sleep.

However, sleep quality may still be affected.

Discomfort, bloating, or anxiety can make it difficult to fall asleep or stay asleep.

Poor sleep, in turn, can worsen symptoms the next day.

This creates a cycle that needs attention.

Emotional Symptoms

IBS affects the mind as well as the body.

You may feel anxious about symptoms, especially in social situations. There may be frustration when plans are disrupted.

Some patients feel embarrassed or misunderstood.

These reactions are natural.

Recognizing them is the first step toward managing them.

Symptoms Outside the Gut

Some patients with IBS also report symptoms outside the digestive system.

These may include:

- Headache
- Back pain
- A general sense of discomfort
- Increased sensitivity to stress

These symptoms reflect the broader effect of IBS on the body.

Variation from Person to Person

No two patients experience IBS in exactly the same way.

Some have mild symptoms. Others have more persistent discomfort.

Symptoms may also change over time.

This variability is normal.

The goal is not to compare yourself with others, but to understand your own pattern.

A Reassuring Thought

Although IBS symptoms can be uncomfortable and sometimes distressing, they do not indicate serious disease.

Understanding this reduces fear and allows you to focus on management.

Chapter Summary

- IBS includes a wide range of symptoms, not just bowel changes
- Abdominal pain often improves after passing stool
- Bloating and gas are common and can be distressing
- Bowel habits may vary between diarrhea and constipation
- Urgency and incomplete evacuation are frequent symptoms
- Mucus may be present, but blood should always be evaluated
- Fatigue and sleep disturbance are common
- Emotional symptoms are part of IBS
- Symptoms vary between individuals and over time

Action Plan

- Continue your symptom diary with more detail
- Note timing of pain, bloating, and bowel movement
- Observe how symptoms relate to meals and stress
- Pay attention to sleep and energy levels
- Focus on patterns rather than individual episodes

CHAPTER 5: When It Is Not IBS – Red Flags and Look-Alike Conditions

Why This Chapter Matters

By now, you have a clear understanding of IBS and its symptoms.

But there is one very important question we must address.

How do we know that these symptoms are truly due to IBS and not something else?

This chapter is not meant to create fear.

It is meant to give you clarity and confidence.

Most people with IBS do not have a serious disease. However, there are certain situations where symptoms may look similar but have a different cause.

Knowing what to watch for helps you stay safe and avoid unnecessary worry.

The Concept of "Red Flags"

Doctors use the term **red flags** to describe symptoms that are not typical of IBS and may require further evaluation.

These symptoms act as warning signs.

If they are present, we need to look deeper.

Important Red Flag Symptoms

You should seek medical attention if you notice any of the following:

- Blood in the stool
- Unexplained weight loss
- Persistent fever
- Anemia (low blood count)
- Symptoms that wake you from sleep regularly
- Severe or progressively worsening abdominal pain
- A family history of colon cancer, inflammatory bowel disease, or celiac disease

Let me emphasize this clearly.

Most patients with IBS do not have these symptoms.

But if they are present, they should never be ignored.

Blood in the Stool

This is one of the most important warning signs.

Blood may appear bright red or darker in color.

IBS does not cause bleeding.

Sometimes the cause may be simple, such as hemorrhoids. But it can also indicate something more serious.

Always get this evaluated.

Unexplained Weight Loss

Weight loss without trying is not typical of IBS.

If you are losing weight without a clear reason, it needs attention.

This may indicate problems with digestion, absorption, or other underlying conditions.

Symptoms That Disturb Sleep

IBS symptoms usually occur during the day.

If you are waking up at night because of diarrhea or pain, this is not typical.

Such symptoms should be evaluated further.

Anemia and Persistent Fatigue

Fatigue is common in IBS, but anemia is not.

If blood tests show anemia, it may indicate blood loss or poor absorption.

This requires further investigation.

Conditions That Can Mimic IBS

Several conditions can produce symptoms similar to IBS.

Understanding them helps avoid confusion and ensures proper care.

Celiac Disease

Celiac disease is a condition in which the body reacts to gluten.

It can cause diarrhea, bloating, fatigue, and weight loss.

Because symptoms overlap with IBS, testing may be recommended in some patients.

Inflammatory Bowel Disease

This includes conditions such as Crohn's disease and ulcerative colitis.

Unlike IBS, these involve inflammation and damage to the intestine.

Symptoms may include diarrhea, abdominal pain, blood in stool, and weight loss.

These conditions require different treatment.

Colon Cancer

This is an important condition to consider, especially in older adults.

Symptoms may include changes in bowel habits, blood in stool, or weight loss.

Routine screening based on age is essential.

Food Intolerance

Some individuals have difficulty digesting certain foods.

Lactose intolerance is common. Some people react to certain carbohydrates.

These can cause bloating, gas, and diarrhea.

Sometimes food intolerance exists along with IBS.

When It Is Not IBS

Concerning Signs and Symptoms

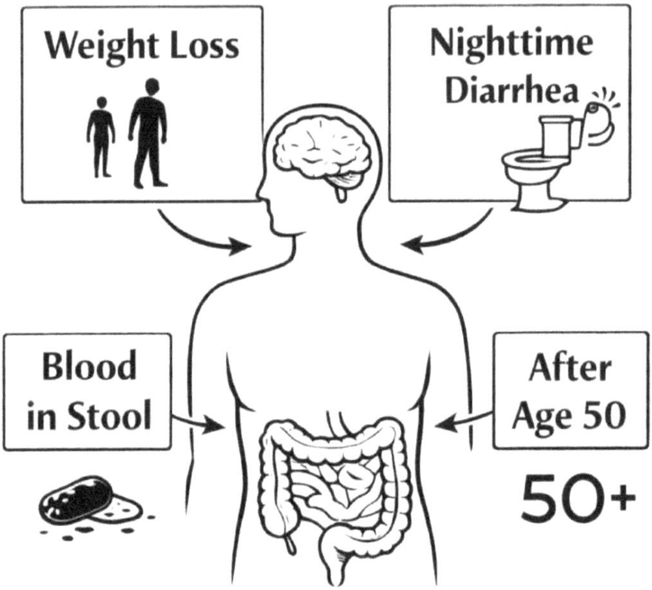

See a *Doctor* for These Symptoms

Small Intestinal Bacterial Overgrowth

In this condition, there is an increased number of bacteria in the small intestine.

Symptoms include bloating, gas, and changes in bowel habits.

It can resemble IBS and may require specific treatment.

Thyroid Disorders

Thyroid function affects bowel movement.

An overactive thyroid may cause diarrhea. An underactive thyroid may cause constipation.

Simple blood tests can help detect these conditions.

Why Proper Evaluation Matters

Evaluation is not about finding something serious.

It is about being sure.

In most cases, after careful assessment, symptoms are due to IBS.

Once serious conditions are ruled out, you can move forward with confidence.

This reassurance is extremely important.

Avoiding Unnecessary Fear

While it is important to be aware of warning signs, it is equally important not to worry unnecessarily.

If your symptoms fit the pattern of IBS and there are no red flags, the likelihood of serious disease is low.

Balanced understanding is the key.

Chapter Summary

- Not all digestive symptoms are due to IBS
- Red flag symptoms require medical evaluation
- Blood in stool, weight loss, anemia, and night symptoms are not typical of IBS
- Several conditions can mimic IBS
- Celiac disease, inflammatory bowel disease, and thyroid disorders are important considerations
- Proper evaluation provides reassurance and ensures safety

Action Plan

- Review your symptoms for any red flags
- Do not ignore warning signs
- Keep track of new or changing symptoms
- Discuss concerns openly with your doctor
- Follow routine screening recommendations

Transition Ahead

Understanding what IBS is not is just as important as understanding what it is.

Now that you know when to seek further evaluation, the next step is to understand how IBS is actually diagnosed in a clear and practical way.

CHAPTER 6: How IBS Is Diagnosed

A Common Concern

One of the most frequent questions patients ask is this:

"Doctor, how do you know this is IBS?"

It is a very reasonable question.

Many people expect that a diagnosis must come from a specific test, a scan, or a lab report.

But IBS is different.

IBS is diagnosed based on **careful understanding of symptoms**, not by a single definitive test.

This often surprises patients.

But once you understand the approach, it becomes logical and reassuring.

IBS Is a Clinical Diagnosis

IBS is what we call a **clinical diagnosis**.

This means it is made based on:

- A detailed history of symptoms

- A pattern that fits well-known criteria
- The absence of warning signs

Doctors listen carefully to what you describe.

The timing of symptoms, their relation to bowel movements, and their duration all provide important clues.

In many cases, this information alone strongly suggests IBS.

The Role of Symptom Patterns

Certain symptom patterns are very typical of IBS.

These include:

- Recurrent abdominal pain
- Pain related to bowel movement
- Changes in stool frequency or consistency
- Symptoms present for several months

When these features are present, the likelihood of IBS is high.

The Rome Criteria

To bring clarity and consistency, doctors use a set of guidelines called the **Rome criteria**.

You do not need to memorize them, but it is helpful to understand the concept.

According to these criteria, IBS is diagnosed when:

- There is recurrent abdominal pain
- The pain occurs at least once a week over a period of time
- It is associated with bowel movement or change in stool pattern

These criteria are based on years of research and help doctors make a confident diagnosis.

Why Tests Are Still Done

If IBS can be diagnosed based on symptoms, why do doctors order tests?

This is an important point.

Tests are not done to prove IBS.

They are done to **rule out other conditions**.

This is especially important if:

- There are red flag symptoms
- The patient is older
- Symptoms are new or changing

Once other conditions are excluded, the diagnosis of IBS becomes clearer and more certain.

Common Tests That May Be Done

Depending on the situation, your doctor may recommend some basic tests.

These may include:

- Blood tests to check for anemia or inflammation
- Tests for celiac disease in selected patients
- Stool tests if infection is suspected
- Thyroid function tests if bowel habits are significantly altered

These tests are usually simple and straightforward.

When Colonoscopy Is Needed

A colonoscopy is not required for every patient with IBS.

However, it may be recommended if:

- You are above a certain age for screening
- There are red flag symptoms
- There is a family history of colon cancer or other bowel diseases

A normal colonoscopy provides strong reassurance.

Avoiding Excessive Testing

Once a proper evaluation has been done and IBS is diagnosed, repeated testing is usually not necessary.

This is very important.

Many patients undergo multiple tests over time, hoping to find a different answer.

In most cases, this does not change the diagnosis.

Instead, it increases anxiety.

Confidence in the diagnosis is a key step in moving forward.

The Importance of Reassurance

A clear diagnosis brings relief.

When you know that there is no serious disease, your focus shifts from fear to management.

This shift is powerful.

It allows you to take control of your symptoms instead of worrying about what might be wrong.

Your Role in the Diagnosis

You play an important role in this process.

The more clearly you describe your symptoms, the easier it is to reach an accurate diagnosis.

Your symptom diary becomes a valuable tool.

It helps your doctor see patterns that may not be obvious in a brief visit.

How IBS Is Diagnosed

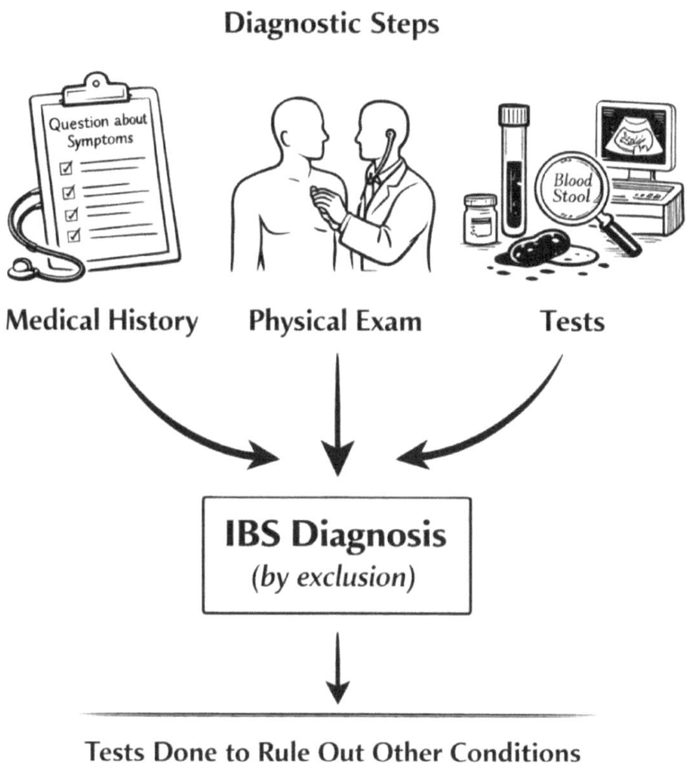

A Balanced Approach

Diagnosis is not about doing every possible test.

It is about doing the **right tests for the right reasons**.

A balanced approach ensures safety without unnecessary procedures.

Chapter Summary

- IBS is diagnosed based on symptoms, not a single test
- It is a clinical diagnosis supported by established criteria
- Tests are used to rule out other conditions
- Basic blood and stool tests may be done
- Colonoscopy is needed only in selected cases
- Excessive testing is usually not helpful
- Reassurance is an important part of diagnosis
- Patient history and symptom patterns are key

Action Plan

- Maintain a clear and honest symptom diary
- Share complete information with your doctor
- Understand that normal test results are reassuring
- Avoid repeated unnecessary testing
- Accept the diagnosis with confidence and move toward management

---

Transition Ahead

Now that you understand how IBS is diagnosed, the next step is to understand why managing it is important.

In the next chapter, we will discuss how IBS can affect your daily life and why taking control early makes a significant difference

CHAPTER 7: Why Treatment Matters – Impact on Daily Life and Long-Term Well-Being

More Than a Digestive Problem

At first glance, IBS may seem like a minor issue.

After all, it does not damage the intestine. It does not lead to cancer. Many patients are told, "Nothing serious is wrong."

While that is medically reassuring, it does not reflect the full reality of living with IBS.

IBS is not dangerous, but it can be deeply disruptive.

It affects how you feel, how you plan your day, how you eat, and how confidently you move through life.

That is why treatment matters.

Not to prevent disease progression, but to restore comfort, confidence, and control.

The Daily Burden of Symptoms

Let us consider a typical day for someone with IBS.

You wake up and wonder how your stomach will behave today.

You think about what to eat, not with enjoyment, but with caution.

If you are going out, you consider where restrooms are located.

If you have an important meeting, you may feel anxious about sudden symptoms.

This constant awareness of your gut can be exhausting.

Even when symptoms are not severe, the uncertainty itself becomes a burden.

The Effect on Work and Productivity

IBS can quietly affect your professional life.

Frequent restroom visits, discomfort during meetings, or reduced concentration due to bloating or pain can impact performance.

Some people avoid travel or important opportunities because of fear of symptoms.

Over time, this can limit growth and confidence.

The Social Impact

Social life is often affected more than people realize.

Eating out becomes stressful. You may avoid certain foods or skip invitations altogether.

Travel can feel risky.

Even simple outings may require planning and caution.

Gradually, this can lead to withdrawal from activities that once brought joy.

The Emotional Toll

Living with IBS can take an emotional toll.

There may be frustration when symptoms interfere with plans. There may be anxiety about when symptoms will occur.

Some patients feel embarrassed discussing bowel-related issues.

Others feel misunderstood when told that "everything is normal."

These emotions are valid.

Recognizing them is the first step toward addressing them.

The Cycle of Symptoms and Stress

IBS often creates a cycle.

Symptoms cause worry. Worry increases stress. Stress worsens symptoms.

This cycle can become self-sustaining.

Breaking this cycle is one of the most important goals of treatment.

And it is very much possible.

Why Ignoring IBS Is Not a Good Strategy

Some patients try to ignore their symptoms.

They hope the problem will go away on its own.

While occasional symptoms may improve, ongoing IBS usually requires a thoughtful approach.

Ignoring it often leads to:

- Continued discomfort
- Increasing frustration
- Unnecessary dietary restrictions
- Reduced quality of life

Addressing IBS early leads to better outcomes.

The Good News: IBS Can Be Managed

Here is the encouraging part.

IBS can be managed effectively.

Not always with a single solution, but with a combination of simple, practical steps.

These include:

- Understanding your pattern
- Making thoughtful dietary changes
- Managing stress in a realistic way
- Using medications when needed

Most patients improve significantly with this approach.

Setting Realistic Expectations

It is important to set realistic goals.

The aim is not perfection.

The aim is control.

You may still have occasional symptoms, but they become less frequent, less intense, and less disruptive.

This shift makes a meaningful difference in daily life.

A Partnership Approach

Managing IBS is a partnership.

You, as the patient, understand your body best.

Your doctor provides guidance and support.

Together, you can develop a plan that works for you.

This personalized approach is key to success.

Taking the First Step

The first step is not a medication.

It is understanding.

Once you understand what is happening in your body, your response changes.

You move from fear to awareness.

From reaction to planning.

This shift alone can improve symptoms.

Chapter Summary

- IBS is not dangerous but can significantly affect daily life
- It impacts work, social life, and emotional well-being
- Symptoms and stress often form a cycle
- Ignoring IBS may worsen quality of life
- IBS can be effectively managed with a structured approach
- The goal is control, not perfection
- A personalized plan works best
- Understanding is the first and most important step

Action Plan

- Reflect on how IBS affects your daily life
- Identify situations that trigger stress or symptoms
- Set realistic goals for improvement
- Begin thinking in terms of management, not cure
- Prepare to take active steps in the next chapters

Transition Ahead

Now that you understand why treatment matters, we move to the most practical part of this journey.

In the next chapter, we will begin with one of the most important and powerful tools in managing IBS.

Your diet.

CHAPTER 8: Diet and IB-Finding What Works for You

A Source of Confusion and Hope

If there is one area where patients feel the most confused, it is diet.

Almost every person with IBS has tried to change their food at some point.

Some eliminate dairy. Others avoid spicy food. Some try gluten-free diets. Many follow advice from friends, family, or the internet.

Sometimes it helps. Often it creates more confusion.

You may begin to wonder:

"What should I eat?"
"What should I avoid?"
"Why does the same food affect me differently on different days?"

These are very real questions.

Let me reassure you from the beginning.

There is no single diet that works for everyone with IBS.

The goal is not to follow a rigid list.

The goal is to understand your own body and make thoughtful, practical choices.

Why Food Affects IBS

Food itself does not cause IBS.

But it can influence symptoms.

This happens for several reasons.

Some foods increase gas production. Some draw more water into the intestine. Some affect the speed of bowel movement.

In IBS, because the gut is more sensitive, these normal effects can feel stronger.

This is why a meal that feels normal for one person may cause discomfort for another.

The Most Common Food Triggers

While individual responses vary, certain foods are commonly associated with symptoms.

These include:

- Gas-producing foods such as beans, cabbage, and onions
- Dairy products in people who are sensitive to lactose
- Fatty or fried foods
- Artificial sweeteners
- Carbonated drinks
- Excess caffeine

It is important to note that these are not "forbidden foods."

They are simply foods to observe and evaluate in your own case.

The Role of Portion Size

Often, it is not just the type of food, but the amount that matters.

A small portion may be well tolerated, while a large portion may trigger symptoms.

This is especially true for foods that produce gas.

Learning portion control is a simple but powerful tool.

Eating Patterns Matter

How you eat is as important as what you eat.

Irregular meals can disturb the natural rhythm of the bowel.

Eating too quickly can increase swallowed air, leading to bloating.

Large, heavy meals may overwhelm the digestive system.

A more balanced approach includes:

- Eating at regular times
- Taking smaller, more frequent meals
- Eating slowly and mindfully

These simple habits can make a noticeable difference.

Diet for IBS: What is FODMAP?

Fermentable sugars that can worsen IBS

F — **Fermentable**

Fermented by gut bacteria

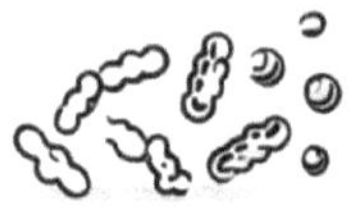

O — **Oligosaccharides**

Fructans, GOS *(grains, some veggies)*

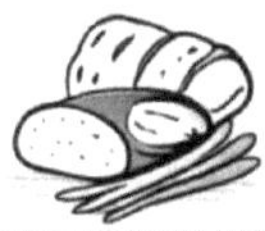

D — **Disaccharides**

Lactose *(milk, dairy)*

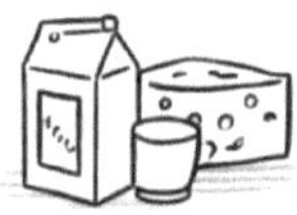

M — **Monosaccharides**

Fructose *(fruit, honey)*

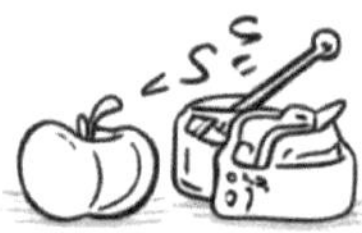

P — **Polyols**

Sorbitol, Mannitol *(sweeteners, stone fruits)*

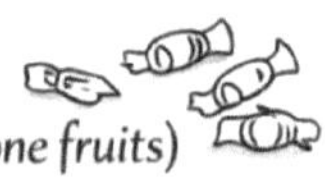

Dietician Can Help Create FODMAP Plan

The Low FODMAP Approach

You may have heard of the **low FODMAP diet**.

This is a structured approach that reduces certain types of carbohydrates that are poorly absorbed and can cause gas and bloating.

Examples include:

- Certain fruits such as apples and pears
- Certain vegetables such as onions and garlic
- Wheat-based products
- Some dairy products

The low FODMAP diet is usually done in phases.

First, certain foods are reduced. Then they are gradually reintroduced to identify triggers.

This approach can be very helpful, but it should be done carefully.

Over-restriction can lead to unnecessary dietary limitations.

Fiber: Friend or Problem

Fiber plays an important role in digestion.

But in IBS, its effects can vary.

There are two types of fiber:

Soluble fiber, found in foods like oats and psyllium, can help regulate bowel movement and is often beneficial.

Insoluble fiber, found in bran and some vegetables, may worsen symptoms in some patients.

The key is gradual adjustment.

Sudden increase in fiber can cause bloating and discomfort.

Hydration

Adequate fluid intake is essential.

Water helps with digestion and stool consistency.

This is especially important for those with constipation.

Avoid excessive intake of carbonated or sugary drinks, as they may worsen symptoms.

Keeping a Food Diary

One of the most effective tools is a simple food diary.

Write down:

- What you eat
- When you eat
- Your symptoms afterward

Over time, patterns begin to emerge.

This helps you make personalized decisions rather than following general advice.

Avoiding Extreme Restrictions

Many patients fall into a common trap.

They begin eliminating more and more foods in an attempt to control symptoms.

This can lead to:

- Nutritional imbalance
- Weight loss
- Increased anxiety around food

A balanced approach is essential.

The goal is to **expand your comfort zone**, not shrink it.

Practical Eating Tips

Some simple habits can make a significant difference:

- Eat slowly and chew food well
- Avoid overeating
- Limit late-night heavy meals
- Be cautious with new or unfamiliar foods
- Maintain regular meal timing

These are small steps, but their impact adds up.

A Flexible Approach

Your diet does not have to be perfect.

It has to be practical and sustainable.

Some days will be better than others.

That is normal.

What matters is the overall pattern, not occasional variations.

Chapter Summary

- There is no single diet for IBS
- Food influences symptoms but does not cause IBS
- Certain foods commonly trigger symptoms
- Portion size and eating habits are important
- The low FODMAP diet may help in selected cases
- Fiber can be helpful but should be adjusted gradually
- Hydration is important
- Food diaries help identify personal triggers
- Avoid overly restrictive diets
- A flexible and balanced approach works best

Action Plan

- Start a detailed food diary
- Observe your response to common trigger foods

- Focus on portion control and regular meal timing
- Increase soluble fiber gradually if needed
- Maintain good hydration
- Avoid unnecessary dietary restrictions
- Begin making small, sustainable changes

Transition Ahead

Diet is a powerful tool, but it is only one part of the picture.

In the next chapter, we will explore another equally important aspect of IBS management.

Your daily habits and lifestyle.

CHAPTER 9: Lifestyle and Daily Habits – Small Changes That Make a Big Difference

Beyond Diet: The Daily Rhythm of Your Body

By now, you have seen how food influences IBS.

But there is another layer that is just as important, and sometimes even more powerful.

Your daily routine.

How you sleep, how you move, how you manage your day, and how you respond to stress all play a role in how your gut behaves.

IBS is not just about what you eat.

It is about how you live.

The encouraging part is this.

Many of these factors are within your control.

Small, steady changes in daily habits can lead to meaningful improvement over time.

The Importance of Routine

The human body thrives on rhythm.

Your digestive system is no exception.

Irregular schedules, skipped meals, and unpredictable routines can disturb the natural pattern of bowel movement.

This may lead to increased symptoms.

Creating a simple, regular routine helps the gut function more smoothly.

Try to:

- Wake up at a consistent time
- Eat meals at regular intervals
- Allow time for bowel movement, especially in the morning

These small adjustments help regulate your internal clock.

Sleep: An Often Overlooked Factor

Sleep has a direct impact on IBS.

Poor sleep can increase sensitivity, worsen pain perception, and affect bowel movement.

Many patients notice that after a restless night, their symptoms feel worse the next day.

Improving sleep does not require complicated steps.

Focus on:

- Going to bed at a regular time
- Reducing screen exposure before sleep
- Keeping your sleeping environment quiet and comfortable

Good sleep supports both the body and the mind.

Physical Activity: A Natural Regulator

Regular physical activity is one of the simplest and most effective ways to improve IBS symptoms.

Movement stimulates the natural rhythm of the intestine.

It can help relieve constipation and reduce stress.

You do not need intense exercise.

Simple activities such as:

- Walking
- Light stretching
- Yoga

can make a noticeable difference.

The key is consistency.

Even 20 to 30 minutes a day can be beneficial.

The Gut–Stress Connection in Daily Life

We discussed earlier how stress affects the gut.

Here, we focus on daily stress.

Modern life is busy and demanding. Completely avoiding stress is not realistic.

But managing your response to stress is possible.

Simple techniques can help calm the nervous system.

These include:

- Slow, deep breathing
- Short breaks during the day
- Spending time in a quiet environment

These are not dramatic changes.

But they gradually reduce the intensity of the gut–brain cycle.

The Role of Mindful Eating

Eating is not just a physical act.

It is also a mental experience.

Eating in a hurry, while distracted, or under stress can affect digestion.

Mindful eating means:

- Sitting down to eat
- Eating slowly

- Paying attention to taste and texture
- Avoiding distractions such as television or phone

This improves digestion and reduces symptoms like bloating.

Hydration and Its Daily Role

You have already learned the importance of hydration.

In daily life, make it a habit rather than an afterthought.

Keep water accessible.

Drink regularly rather than waiting until you feel thirsty.

This is especially helpful for those with constipation.

Managing Travel and Busy Days

Many patients worry about symptoms when traveling or during busy schedules.

Planning helps reduce anxiety.

Some practical steps include:

- Knowing restroom locations in advance
- Carrying simple, familiar snacks
- Avoiding large or unfamiliar meals
- Staying hydrated

Preparation reduces uncertainty.

And reducing uncertainty reduces stress.

Breaking the Cycle of Overthinking

One common challenge in IBS is over-focusing on symptoms.

Every small sensation may be noticed and analyzed.

This can increase anxiety and worsen symptoms.

It is important to find a balance.

Be aware of your body, but do not become overly focused on every detail.

Gradually shift attention toward normal activities and routines.

Building Confidence Over Time

Improvement in IBS is gradual.

It comes from consistent, small steps.

Each positive change builds confidence.

Confidence reduces fear.

And when fear reduces, symptoms often improve.

This is an important and encouraging cycle.

Diet & Lifestyle Changes That Work

Helpful Strategies

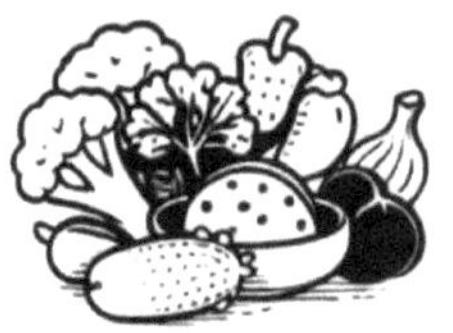

Low FODMAP Diet

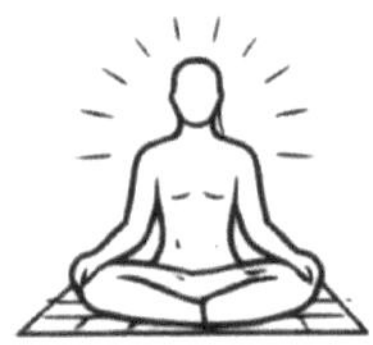

Reduce Stress

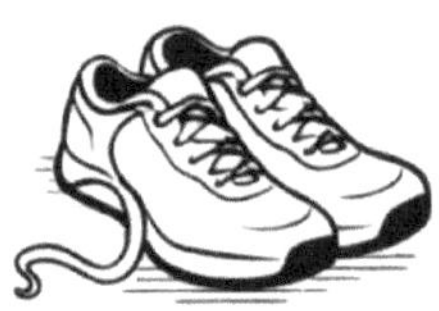

Exercise Regularly

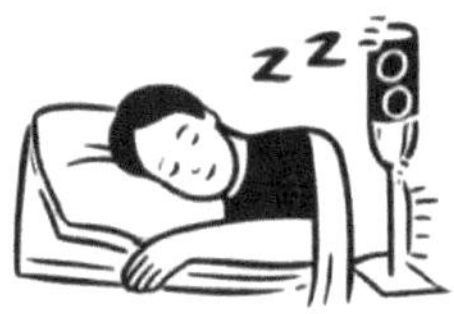

Adequate Sleep

Effective Ways to Manage IBS

A Practical Approach

You do not need to change everything at once.

Choose a few habits and work on them steadily.

Consistency matters more than perfection.

Chapter Summary

- Daily routine plays a major role in IBS
- Regular sleep improves symptom control
- Physical activity helps bowel movement and reduces stress
- Stress management reduces symptom intensity
- Mindful eating improves digestion
- Hydration is essential
- Planning helps manage travel and busy days
- Avoid over-focusing on symptoms
- Small, consistent changes lead to improvement

Action Plan

- Establish a regular daily routine
- Improve sleep habits
- Begin a simple daily exercise routine
- Practice slow breathing or relaxation techniques
- Eat meals calmly and without distraction
- Stay well hydrated
- Prepare ahead for travel or busy days
- Focus on steady improvement rather than perfection

Transition Ahead

So far, we have focused on understanding IBS, diet, and lifestyle.

Now we move to another important area.

In the next chapter, we will discuss medications.

Not as a first step, but as a useful support when needed.

CHAPTER 10: Medications for IBS – When and How to Use Them Wisely

A Balanced View of Medications

By this point, you have learned that diet and lifestyle form the foundation of IBS management.

However, there are times when symptoms persist despite these efforts.

This is where medications can help.

It is important to approach this topic with balance.

Medications are not a cure for IBS. But they can reduce symptoms, improve comfort, and help you regain control of your daily life.

The goal is not to depend on medicines unnecessarily, but to use them thoughtfully when needed.

Why Medications Are Needed

IBS symptoms arise from multiple factors:

- Irregular bowel movement
- Increased gut sensitivity
- Changes in gut–brain communication

Medications target one or more of these mechanisms.

Some help regulate bowel movement. Others reduce pain or bloating. Some act on the nervous system to reduce sensitivity.

Choosing the right medication depends on your symptoms.

Treating Constipation

For patients with constipation-predominant IBS, the goal is to improve stool movement and ease passage.

Common options include:

Fiber supplements
Soluble fiber such as psyllium can help regulate bowel movement. It should be introduced gradually.

Osmotic laxatives
These help draw water into the stool, making it softer and easier to pass.

Prescription medications
Certain newer medications improve bowel movement by increasing fluid secretion or enhancing motility.

These are used when simpler measures are not enough.

Treating Diarrhea

For patients with diarrhea-predominant IBS, the aim is to slow bowel movement and reduce urgency.

Options include:

Anti-diarrheal medications
These reduce stool frequency and improve control.

Bile acid binders
In some patients, excess bile acids contribute to diarrhea. These medications can help.

Prescription medications
Some drugs act directly on the intestine to reduce diarrhea and improve symptoms.

Treating Abdominal Pain and Cramping

Pain is one of the most distressing symptoms of IBS.

Several approaches can help:

Antispasmodic medications
These relax the muscles of the intestine and reduce cramping.

Peppermint oil
A natural option that may reduce muscle spasm and discomfort.

Low-dose antidepressants
These are used not for depression, but to reduce gut sensitivity and pain perception.

They work by modifying how the brain processes signals from the intestine.

Managing Bloating and Gas

Bloating can be particularly uncomfortable.

Options include:

- Dietary adjustments
- Medications that reduce gas formation
- In selected cases, antibiotics that target gut bacteria

These approaches are chosen based on individual symptoms.

The Role of Probiotics

Probiotics are beneficial bacteria that may help restore balance in the gut.

Some patients experience improvement in bloating and overall symptoms.

However, results vary.

Not all probiotics work the same way.

A trial of a specific product for a few weeks may help determine benefit.

Treating the Gut–Brain Axis

Because IBS involves the interaction between the gut and brain, some treatments focus on this connection.

Low-dose antidepressants and certain newer medications can help reduce sensitivity and improve overall symptom control.

This does not mean that IBS is a psychological condition.

It means that the gut–brain communication can be adjusted for better balance.

Avoiding Overuse of Medications

It is important not to rely excessively on medications.

Frequent switching or combining multiple drugs without a clear plan can lead to confusion and side effects.

A structured approach works best.

Use medications:

- When symptoms are significant
- In combination with lifestyle changes
- Under proper guidance

Personalizing Treatment

There is no single medication that works for everyone.

Treatment must be tailored.

Some patients need occasional support. Others may need longer-term management.

Regular follow-up and adjustment help achieve the best results.

Safety and Side Effects

All medications have potential side effects.

Most IBS medications are safe when used appropriately.

However, it is important to:

- Follow prescribed doses
- Report any unusual symptoms
- Avoid self-medication without guidance

A Practical Perspective

Think of medications as tools.

They are there to help you when needed.

But the foundation of long-term improvement remains:

- Understanding your condition
- Managing diet and lifestyle
- Reducing stress

When these are in place, medications become more effective.

Medicines for IBS

Common Treatments and Medications

F

Antispasmodics

Eases abdominal cramping; relaxes gut muscles

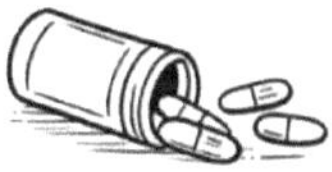

Antidiarrheals

Helps reduce diarrhea and frequent loose stools

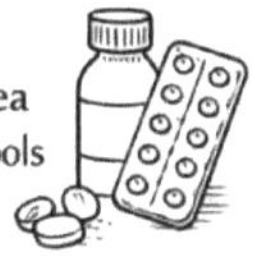

L

Laxatives

Alleviates constipation; helps with regularity

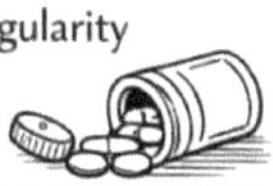

Fiber Supplements

Improves bowel movement consistency

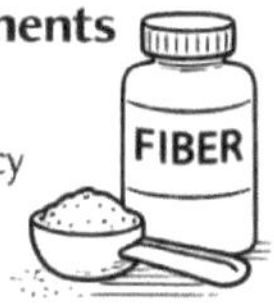

D

Probiotics

Supports gut health; promotes healthy bacteria

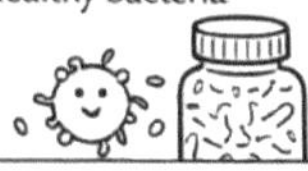

Pain Relievers

Helps relieve stomach pain and discomfort

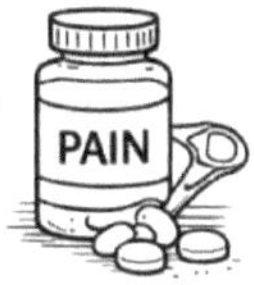

How the Low FODMAP Diet Works

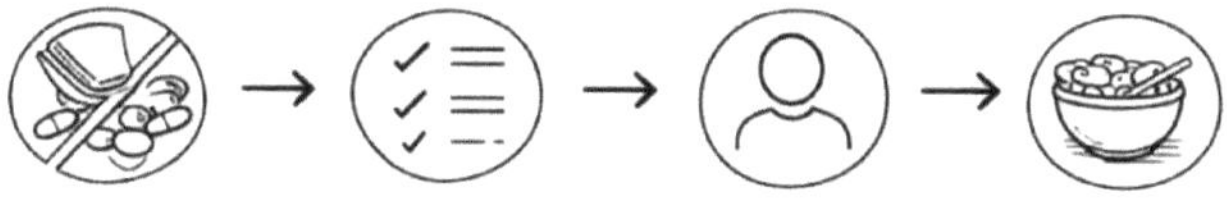

1. **Elimination** — Avoid Nigh FODMAP foods for 2–6 weeks.
2. **Reintroduction** — Reintroduce FODMAPs one group at a time.
3. **Personalization** — identify your triggers and tolerance levels.
4. **Pain Relievers** — Follow a balanced diet that works for you.

⚠ **Important:** Consult a healthcare provider to choose the right medication and dosage. Other prescriptions, such as antidepressants or antibiotics, may be recommended for severe or specific cases of IBS.

Chapter Summary

- Medications help manage symptoms but do not cure IBS
- Treatment depends on symptom pattern
- Constipation, diarrhea, pain, and bloating are treated differently
- Probiotics may help in some patients
- Some medications act on the gut–brain connection
- Overuse of medications should be avoided
- Treatment should be personalized
- Safety and proper use are important

Action Plan

- Identify your main symptoms
- Discuss appropriate medication options with your doctor
- Use medications as part of a broader plan
- Avoid frequent changes without guidance
- Monitor response and side effects
- Continue lifestyle and dietary measures

Transition Ahead

Medications are helpful, but they are only one part of a complete approach.

There are also non-medication therapies that can significantly improve IBS symptoms.

In the next chapter, we will explore these approaches and how they fit into your overall plan.

CHAPTER 11: Non-Medication Therapies – Calming the Gut–Brain Connection

Looking Beyond Medicines

By now, you have seen that medications can help when symptoms are troubling.

But there is another powerful area of treatment that often receives less attention.

Non-medication therapies.

These approaches do not work by directly changing the bowel. Instead, they help regulate the **gut–brain connection**, which, as you now understand, plays a central role in IBS.

For many patients, these methods bring meaningful and lasting improvement.

Why These Therapies Work

IBS is not simply a problem of the intestine.

It involves how the brain and gut communicate.

When this communication becomes overactive or unbalanced, symptoms appear.

Non-medication therapies help:

- Reduce sensitivity of the gut
- Calm the nervous system
- Break the cycle of stress and symptoms

They are not alternatives to medical care.

They are an essential part of a complete, well-rounded approach.

Understanding the Mind–Body Connection

Let us be very clear.

When we talk about the mind–body connection, we are not saying that IBS is "in your head."

We are saying that your body responds to signals from your brain.

Just as stress can increase heart rate or blood pressure, it can also affect digestion.

When you understand this, it becomes easier to work with your body rather than against it.

Cognitive Behavioral Therapy

Cognitive behavioral therapy, often called CBT, is one of the most studied approaches for IBS.

It focuses on identifying and modifying patterns of thinking and behavior that may worsen symptoms.

For example:

- Fear of symptoms can increase anxiety
- Anxiety can worsen gut sensitivity
- This increases symptoms further

CBT helps break this cycle.

It teaches practical ways to respond differently to symptoms and reduce their impact.

Gut-Directed Hypnotherapy

This may sound unusual at first, but it is a well-recognized therapy for IBS.

Gut-directed hypnotherapy uses guided relaxation and focused attention to influence gut function.

It helps reduce sensitivity and improve symptom control.

Many patients report significant improvement with this approach.

It is gentle, non-invasive, and increasingly used in IBS management.

Relaxation Techniques

Simple relaxation methods can be surprisingly effective.

These include:

- Slow, deep breathing
- Progressive muscle relaxation
- Quiet time away from stimulation

These techniques reduce the body's stress response.

With regular practice, they help calm the gut.

Mindfulness and Awareness

Mindfulness means paying attention to the present moment without judgment.

In IBS, this helps reduce the tendency to react strongly to symptoms.

Instead of immediately worrying or anticipating the worst, you observe the sensation calmly.

Over time, this reduces the intensity of the gut–brain cycle.

Yoga and Gentle Movement

Yoga combines physical movement, breathing, and relaxation.

It improves flexibility, reduces stress, and supports digestion.

Even simple stretches can relieve tension in the abdomen and improve comfort.

Regular practice can be very beneficial.

The Role of Counseling

For some patients, ongoing stress, anxiety, or life challenges contribute to symptoms.

Talking to a trained counselor can help.

This is not about labeling IBS as a psychological condition.

It is about addressing factors that influence how your body responds.

Support in this area can make a meaningful difference.

Building a Personalized Plan

Not every therapy works for everyone.

Some patients respond well to relaxation techniques. Others benefit more from structured therapy such as CBT.

The key is to explore what works for you.

Start with simple methods.

If needed, consider more structured approaches.

Consistency Matters

These therapies do not work overnight.

They require regular practice.

But the results are often long-lasting.

Unlike medications, which act quickly but temporarily, these approaches gradually change how your body responds.

This leads to more stable improvement.

Removing the Stigma

Some patients hesitate to try these approaches.

They feel it implies that their condition is psychological.

That is not true.

These therapies are part of modern, evidence-based care for IBS.

They address the real biological connection between the brain and the gut.

A Practical Perspective

Think of these methods as tools to retrain your system.

They help your body return to a more balanced and less reactive state.

Used along with diet, lifestyle changes, and medications when needed, they form a complete approach.

Chapter Summary

- IBS involves the gut–brain connection
- Non-medication therapies help regulate this connection
- CBT can reduce symptom-related anxiety and improve control
- Gut-directed hypnotherapy is an effective option
- Relaxation and mindfulness reduce stress response
- Yoga supports both body and mind
- Counseling can help address underlying stress
- Consistency is key to success
- These approaches are evidence-based and important

Action Plan

- Begin with simple daily relaxation exercises
- Practice slow, deep breathing for a few minutes each day
- Try mindful awareness of symptoms without reacting
- Consider yoga or gentle stretching
- Explore structured therapy if symptoms persist
- Be consistent and patient with these methods

Transition Ahead

You now have a comprehensive understanding of treatment options.

In the next chapter, we will bring everything together into a clear, practical plan that you can follow in your daily life.

CHAPTER 12: A Practical Plan of Action – Taking Control Step by Step

Bringing Everything Together

You have now traveled through the most important aspects of IBS.

You understand what it is, how it develops, how it is diagnosed, and how it can be managed through diet, lifestyle, medications, and non-medication therapies.

Now comes the most important part.

Putting it all together in a way that works in your daily life.

This chapter is about creating a **simple, practical, and realistic plan** that you can follow without feeling overwhelmed.

Because real improvement in IBS does not come from knowing everything.

It comes from applying a few important things consistently.

Step One: Understand Your Pattern

Before you make changes, take a moment to understand your own pattern.

Ask yourself:

- Do I have more constipation or diarrhea?
- When are my symptoms worse?
- Are they related to meals, stress, or routine?

Your symptom diary will help you answer these questions.

This step gives direction to everything that follows.

Step Two: Start with Diet

Do not try to change everything at once.

Begin with a few simple adjustments:

- Eat at regular times
- Reduce large, heavy meals
- Identify and limit obvious trigger foods
- Increase soluble fiber gradually if needed

If symptoms persist, consider a structured approach such as a low FODMAP plan under guidance.

Remember, the goal is not restriction.

The goal is balance.

Step Three: Build a Daily Routine

Your gut responds to rhythm.

Try to:

- Wake up at a consistent time
- Eat meals regularly
- Allow time for bowel movement, especially in the morning

These small habits help regulate your digestive system.

Step Four: Improve Sleep

Good sleep supports the entire system.

Make it a priority.

- Maintain a regular sleep schedule
- Reduce screen time before bed
- Create a calm sleeping environment

Better sleep often leads to better symptom control.

Step Five: Stay Physically Active

Movement supports digestion and reduces stress.

You do not need intense exercise.

Start with:

- Daily walking
- Light stretching
- Gentle yoga

Consistency is more important than intensity.

Step Six: Manage Stress in a Practical Way

You do not need to eliminate stress.

You need to respond to it differently.

Begin with simple techniques:

- Slow, deep breathing
- Short periods of quiet time
- Stepping away from stressful situations when possible

Over time, this reduces the impact of stress on your gut.

Step Seven: Use Medications Thoughtfully

If symptoms are significant, medications can help.

Use them as part of your plan, not as the only solution.

- Match the medication to your main symptom
- Avoid frequent changes without guidance
- Monitor your response

Medications work best when combined with lifestyle measures.

Step Eight: Consider Non-Medication Therapies

If symptoms persist or stress plays a major role, consider additional support.

- Relaxation techniques
- Cognitive behavioral therapy
- Mindfulness practices

These approaches help calm the gut–brain connection.

Step Nine: Avoid Common Mistakes

Many patients unintentionally make their symptoms worse.

Avoid:

- Constantly changing diets
- Eliminating too many foods
- Over-focusing on symptoms
- Repeating unnecessary tests

A steady, balanced approach works best.

Step Ten: Track Progress, Not Perfection

IBS does not improve in a straight line.

There will be good days and difficult days.

Do not judge your progress based on one day.

Look at overall trends.

Small improvements add up.

A Weekly Plan Example

To make things more practical, here is a simple weekly approach:

- Focus on regular meals and hydration
- Maintain daily physical activity
- Practice relaxation techniques for a few minutes each day
- Review your symptom diary at the end of the week
- Make small adjustments based on patterns

This keeps the process manageable.

Building Confidence Over Time

As you follow your plan, something important happens.

You begin to understand your body.

You recognize patterns.

You respond calmly instead of reacting with fear.

This builds confidence.

And confidence itself reduces symptoms.

When to Seek Help

Even with a good plan, you may need guidance at times.

Seek help if:

- Symptoms are not improving
- New symptoms appear
- You feel uncertain or anxious

Working with your doctor helps refine your plan.

A Simple Truth

There is no single solution for IBS.

But there is a clear path.

Understanding, patience, and consistency lead to improvement.

Chapter Summary

- A structured plan makes IBS manageable
- Start by understanding your symptom pattern
- Make gradual dietary changes
- Build a regular daily routine
- Improve sleep and stay active
- Manage stress in practical ways
- Use medications wisely when needed
- Avoid common mistakes
- Focus on progress over perfection

- Confidence grows with consistency

Action Plan

- Create your personal IBS management plan
- Start with 2 to 3 small changes this week
- Continue your symptom and food diary
- Practice relaxation daily
- Review progress weekly
- Stay patient and consistent

Transition Ahead

You now have a clear and practical plan.

In the next chapter, we will look beyond short-term control and focus on maintaining long-term well-being and confidence with IBS.

CHAPTER 13: Living Well with IBS - Long-Term Control and Confidence

A Shift in Perspective

By now, you have learned a great deal about IBS.

You understand the condition, its causes, its symptoms, and the many ways to manage it.

But there is one final and very important step.

Learning how to **live well with IBS** over the long term.

This is where your mindset begins to change.

You move from trying to "fix a problem" to learning how to **work with your body**.

That shift makes all the difference.

IBS Is a Long-Term Condition

IBS is not something that appears one day and disappears the next.

It tends to follow a long-term course.

Symptoms may come and go. There may be periods when you feel almost normal, and other times when symptoms return.

This pattern is typical.

Understanding this prevents unnecessary frustration.

Your goal is not to eliminate every symptom forever.

Your goal is to **reduce the impact of symptoms on your life**.

Recognizing Flare-Ups

Most patients with IBS experience flare-ups.

These are periods when symptoms become more noticeable.

Flare-ups may be triggered by:

- Changes in diet
- Stressful situations
- Travel or changes in routine
- Illness or lack of sleep

Recognizing these triggers helps you respond calmly.

Instead of feeling alarmed, you understand that this is part of the condition.

Managing Flare-Ups Calmly

When symptoms increase, your response matters.

A calm, structured approach works best.

Return to your basics:

- Simplify your diet temporarily
- Maintain hydration
- Use medications if needed
- Practice relaxation techniques

Avoid drastic changes.

Flare-ups usually settle with time and steady management.

Building Long-Term Habits

The most successful patients are not those who try everything at once.

They are those who build simple habits and maintain them.

These include:

- Regular meals
- Consistent sleep
- Daily physical activity
- Stress management

These habits create stability.

And stability reduces symptoms.

Maintaining Flexibility

Life is not always predictable.

There will be occasions when your routine changes.

Travel, social events, and busy schedules are part of life.

You do not need to avoid them.

Instead, you learn to adapt.

With experience, you will know:

- Which foods are safer choices
- How to plan ahead
- How to manage symptoms if they occur

This flexibility allows you to live fully.

Confidence Comes from Experience

At the beginning, IBS may feel overwhelming.

You may worry about every meal or outing.

But over time, something changes.

You begin to understand your body.

You recognize patterns.

You respond more calmly.

This builds confidence.

And with confidence, symptoms often become less disruptive.

Avoiding the Trap of Perfection

One common mistake is trying to achieve perfect control.

This is not realistic.

Even with the best plan, occasional symptoms will occur.

Do not see this as failure.

See it as part of the journey.

A balanced approach leads to better long-term results.

Staying Informed, Not Overwhelmed

There is a lot of information available about IBS.

Some of it is helpful. Some of it is confusing.

Be selective.

Focus on reliable, practical advice.

Avoid constantly changing your approach based on new trends.

Consistency is more important than constant experimentation.

The Role of Follow-Up

Regular follow-up with your doctor can be helpful.

It allows for:

- Adjustment of treatment
- Addressing new concerns
- Reinforcing effective strategies

You do not have to manage everything alone.

Supporting Your Overall Health

IBS management is part of a larger goal.

Your overall health.

Pay attention to:

- Balanced nutrition
- Regular activity
- Emotional well-being

When your general health improves, your IBS often improves as well.

A Positive Outlook

It is important to end this journey on a positive note.

IBS can be challenging, but it is manageable.

Most patients improve significantly over time.

With understanding and steady effort, you can lead a comfortable and active life.

Chapter Summary

- IBS is a long-term condition with variable symptoms
- Flare-ups are common and usually manageable
- Simple habits provide long-term stability
- Flexibility allows you to live normally
- Confidence grows with experience
- Perfection is not necessary
- Consistency is more important than constant change
- Regular follow-up supports long-term success
- Overall health plays an important role

Action Plan

- Accept IBS as a manageable long-term condition
- Identify your common triggers for flare-ups
- Develop a simple plan for managing flare-ups
- Maintain healthy daily habits
- Stay flexible during travel and social situations
- Avoid overreacting to occasional symptoms
- Continue learning in a balanced way
- Follow up with your doctor when needed

Moving Forward

You now have the knowledge, the tools, and the perspective needed to manage IBS effectively.

The next and final section will bring everything together and leave you with a clear, confident path forward.

CHAPTER 14: Common Myths and Misconceptions About IBS

Why Myths Matter

In my years of practice, I have noticed something very important.

Many patients suffer not only from IBS, but also from **wrong beliefs about IBS**.

These misconceptions create unnecessary fear, confusion, and frustration.

Some patients restrict their diet too much. Others worry about serious disease despite normal tests. Some feel that their condition is not being taken seriously.

Clearing these myths is an essential step in your journey.

When you replace confusion with clarity, your approach becomes calmer and more effective.

Myth 1: IBS Is Not a Real Disease

This is one of the most common and harmful misconceptions.

Some people believe that if tests are normal, the problem must not be real.

This is not true.

IBS is a well-recognized medical condition. It has been studied extensively. The symptoms arise from real changes in gut function and sensitivity.

The fact that it does not show up on routine tests does not make it less real.

Your symptoms are valid.

Myth 2: IBS Is "All in the Mind"

Many patients are told that their symptoms are due to stress or anxiety.

This can feel dismissive.

The truth is more balanced.

Stress can influence IBS, but it does not create the condition by itself.

IBS involves a complex interaction between the gut and the brain.

So while the mind plays a role, the condition is not imaginary.

It is a physical condition with real biological mechanisms.

Myth 3: IBS Will Turn Into a Serious Disease

This is a common fear.

Patients worry that IBS may eventually lead to cancer or other serious problems.

Let me reassure you clearly.

IBS does not cause cancer. It does not damage the intestine.

Once serious conditions have been ruled out, IBS remains a benign condition.

Understanding this reduces fear and anxiety.

Myth 4: You Must Avoid Many Foods

Many patients begin eliminating food after food in an attempt to control symptoms.

Over time, their diet becomes very limited.

This is not necessary.

While certain foods may trigger symptoms, most patients can tolerate a wide variety of foods with proper adjustment.

The goal is not restriction.

The goal is understanding and moderation.

Myth 5: There Is One Perfect Diet for IBS

There is no universal IBS diet.

What works for one person may not work for another.

The low FODMAP diet can be helpful, but even that is not a permanent restriction.

Personalization is key.

Learning your own triggers is more important than following a fixed list.

Myth 6: Medications Alone Can Solve the Problem

Some patients expect a single medication to eliminate all symptoms.

This is rarely the case.

IBS management requires a combination of:

- Diet
- Lifestyle
- Stress management
- Medications when needed

Medications are helpful, but they are only one part of the plan.

Myth 7: You Must Live With Constant Discomfort

Another misconception is that IBS cannot be improved.

This is not true.

While IBS may not disappear completely, symptoms can be significantly reduced.

Many patients achieve good control and lead comfortable lives.

Improvement is realistic and achievable.

Myth 8: Frequent Testing Will Find the Answer

Patients sometimes feel that repeated testing will eventually reveal the cause.

In most cases, once proper evaluation is done, further testing does not change the diagnosis.

Instead, it increases anxiety.

Confidence in the diagnosis allows you to focus on management.

Myth 9: IBS Is the Same in Everyone

IBS varies from person to person.

Symptoms, triggers, and responses to treatment differ.

Comparing yourself with others can lead to confusion.

Your plan should be based on your own experience.

Myth 10: Improvement Must Be Quick

Many patients expect rapid improvement.

When symptoms persist, they feel discouraged.

IBS improves gradually.

It requires patience and consistency.

Small changes over time lead to meaningful results.

A Clear Perspective

When these myths are removed, something important happens.

You begin to see IBS clearly.

Not as a mysterious or frightening condition, but as a manageable one.

Clarity reduces fear.

And reduced fear improves symptoms.

Chapter Summary

- IBS is a real and well-recognized condition
- It is not "all in the mind"
- It does not lead to serious disease
- Extreme dietary restriction is not necessary

- There is no single diet for everyone
- Medications alone are not enough
- Symptoms can be improved significantly
- Repeated testing is usually not helpful
- IBS varies between individuals
- Improvement takes time and consistency

Action Plan

- Identify and challenge your own misconceptions
- Avoid unnecessary dietary restrictions
- Focus on balanced, practical changes
- Accept gradual improvement
- Build confidence in your management plan
- Stay consistent with your approach

Moving Ahead

With a clear understanding and the right mindset, you are now ready to bring everything together and move forward with confidence.

In the final chapter, we will summarize your journey and leave you with a clear, reassuring message for the future.

CHAPTER 15: Moving Forward – A Clear Path to Living Well with IBS

Looking Back at Your Journey

You have come a long way.

When you began this book, IBS may have felt confusing, unpredictable, and even overwhelming. You may have had many unanswered questions and perhaps some worries.

Now, you have clarity.

You understand what IBS is, how it develops, and why symptoms occur. You know how diet, lifestyle, stress, and the gut–brain connection all play a role. You have learned practical steps, not just theory.

This understanding is powerful.

Because when you understand your body, you are no longer reacting with fear.

You are responding with confidence.

A New Way of Thinking

The most important change is not just what you do.

It is how you think.

Instead of asking, "Why is this happening to me?" You begin to ask, "How can I manage this better?"

This shift reduces anxiety.

It allows you to focus on solutions rather than problems.

And that alone begins to improve your symptoms.

Your Personal Plan Matters Most

There is no single solution that works for everyone.

Your plan is your own.

It is built from:

- Your symptom pattern
- Your dietary responses
- Your lifestyle
- Your stress triggers

What matters is not perfection.

What matters is consistency.

Small Steps, Real Results

IBS does not improve with one big change.

It improves with small, steady steps.

Regular meals.
Better sleep.
A short daily walk.
A few minutes of relaxation.

These may seem simple.

But together, they create a strong foundation.

Over time, these small steps lead to meaningful improvement.

Handling Difficult Days

There will be days when symptoms return.

This is normal.

It does not mean that your plan has failed.

It simply means that your body is responding to temporary changes.

On such days:

- Stay calm
- Return to your routine
- Simplify your diet
- Use medications if needed

Symptoms usually settle.

Your response makes the difference.

Confidence Changes Everything

At the beginning, IBS may have controlled your life.

Now, you begin to take control.

You understand your triggers.

You know how to respond.

You are no longer guessing.

This builds confidence.

And confidence reduces the impact of symptoms.

Living Fully, Not Carefully

One of the biggest goals in managing IBS is this:

To live your life fully. Not cautiously.

You should be able to:

- Enjoy meals
- Travel with reasonable planning
- Participate in social activities
- Focus on your work and interests

IBS should not define your life.

It should become just one part of your health, not the center of it.

Living Well with IBS

Helpful Tips for Managing Irritable Bowel Syndrome

Follow a Low FODMAP Diet

Work with a dietitian to identify & avoid trigger foods

Exercise Regularly

Aim for at least 30 minutes of moderate activity most days

L

Aim for at least 30 minutes of moderate activity most days

Manage Stress

Practice relaxation techniques like medit-ation or deep breathing

Establish Routine

Eat meals and use the bathroom at regular times

Get Enough Sleep

Aim for 7-9 hours of quality sleep per night

Avoid Gas-Producing Foods

Limit beans, lentils, carbonated drinks, and cruciferous vegetables

Limit Caffeine, Alcohol

Consume with caution; can worsen IBS symptoms

Eat Small, Frequent Meals

Helps reduce bloating and discomfort

Take Medications as Directed

Follow your doctor's guidance on IBS medications

See a Doctor for Severe or Persistent Symptoms

If you experience severe, persistent, or unusual **symptoms** (bleeding, weight loss, severe pain), seek medical care.

When You Need Support

You do not have to manage everything alone.

If symptoms change or become difficult, seek guidance.

A doctor can help refine your plan.

Sometimes, just a small adjustment makes a big difference.

A Final Reassuring Message

Let me leave you with a clear and honest message.

IBS is real.

It can be uncomfortable and sometimes frustrating.

But it is not dangerous.

And most importantly, it is manageable.

With understanding, patience, and steady effort, you can live a comfortable, confident, and active life.

Chapter Summary

- You now understand IBS clearly
- A change in mindset is essential
- Your management plan should be personalized
- Small, consistent steps lead to improvement

- Flare-ups are normal and manageable
- Confidence reduces symptom impact
- IBS should not limit your life
- Support is available when needed
- Long-term improvement is achievable

Action Plan

- Continue following your personalized plan
- Focus on consistency rather than perfection
- Respond calmly to flare-ups
- Maintain healthy habits
- Stay confident in your ability to manage IBS
- Seek help when needed

Final Thought

Take a moment to reflect.

You now have the knowledge and tools that many patients search for over years.

Use them wisely.

Move forward with confidence.

And most importantly, live your life fully and freely.

APPENDIX A: A Simple IBS-Friendly Meal Guide

A Practical Way to Eat Without Fear

Diet in IBS can feel confusing.

Instead of long lists of what to avoid, let us keep it simple and practical.

The goal is to help you eat comfortably, not restrict unnecessarily.

Foods That Are Generally Well Tolerated

These foods are usually easier on the digestive system:

- Rice, oats, and simple grains
- Cooked vegetables such as carrots, spinach, zucchini
- Lean proteins such as chicken, fish, eggs
- Yogurt (if tolerated)
- Bananas and some berries
- Plain bread or toast

These can form the base of your daily meals.

Foods to Be Careful With

These foods may trigger symptoms in some people:

- Beans and lentils
- Onions and garlic
- Fried or fatty foods
- Carbonated drinks
- Artificial sweeteners
- Excess caffeine

You do not need to avoid them completely.

Observe your response.

A Sample Day

Breakfast
Oatmeal with a banana and a cup of tea

Lunch
Rice with cooked vegetables and grilled chicken

Evening snack
Yogurt or a small handful of nuts

Dinner
Light meal with soup, vegetables, and simple protein

Keep meals simple and balanced.

Key Message

Eat calmly, eat regularly, and observe your body.

APPENDIX B: Fiber Guide for IBS

Understanding Fiber

Fiber is helpful, but it must be used wisely.

Soluble Fiber (Usually Helpful)

- Oats
- Psyllium
- Apples (in small amounts)
- Carrots

These can help regulate bowel movement.

Insoluble Fiber (May Cause Symptoms)

- Wheat bran
- Raw vegetables
- Some whole grains

These may worsen bloating in some patients.

How to Use Fiber

- Increase gradually

- Drink adequate water
- Observe your response

Key Message

Start slow. Adjust based on your body's response.

APPENDIX C: Symptom and Food Diary Template

Why This Helps

A simple diary can reveal patterns that are otherwise missed.

What to Record

Date
Time of meal
Food eaten
Symptoms
Stress level
Bowel movement details

Example Entry

Morning
Oatmeal and tea
Mild bloating

Lunch
Rice and vegetables
No symptoms

Evening
Fried food
Increased discomfort

Key Message

Patterns guide better decisions.

APPENDIX D: Quick Relaxation Techniques

Simple Methods That Work

You do not need long sessions.

A few minutes can help.

Deep Breathing

- Sit comfortably
- Inhale slowly through the nose
- Exhale gently
- Repeat for 5 minutes

Muscle Relaxation

- Tighten one muscle group
- Hold briefly
- Release slowly

Quiet Time

- Sit in a calm place
- Focus on your breathing
- Let thoughts pass without reacting

APPENDIX E: When to See a Doctor Again

Important Situations

Seek medical advice if you notice:

- Blood in stool
- Unexplained weight loss
- Persistent or worsening symptoms
- New symptoms after age 50
- Ongoing diarrhea at night

Routine Follow-Up

Even if symptoms are stable, periodic review can help refine your plan.

Key Message

Stay alert, but do not worry unnecessarily.

APPENDIX F: A Simple Weekly IBS Plan

Keep It Practical

Do not try to do everything at once.

Weekly Focus

- Maintain regular meals
- Stay hydrated
- Exercise at least 5 days a week
- Practice relaxation daily
- Review your symptom diary

End of Week Reflection

- What improved
- What triggered symptoms
- What small change to try next week

Key Message

Small weekly improvements lead to long-term success.

FINAL NOTE

This book was written to guide you, not to overwhelm you.

If you remember just a few things, let them be these:

- IBS is real, but not dangerous
- Understanding reduces fear
- Small, steady steps bring improvement
- Your body can be guided toward balance

Take your time.

Stay patient.

And trust the process.

Thank You and Please Review the Book

Thank you for taking the time to read this book. I sincerely hope it has helped you understand your health a little more clearly and has given you practical, everyday steps you can follow with confidence. If you found this book helpful, **I would truly appreciate it if you could leave a brief and honest review.** Even a few lines sharing your experience can make a meaningful difference. Your feedback helps other readers find reliable, trustworthy health information and supports them in making better decisions for themselves and their families.

Warm regards,
Dr Prabhat Das

Continue your Healthcare Journey

Good health is a journey, not a single step. It is not achieved in one day or with one book. That is why I created the "Better Health with Dr Das" series, with each book addressing a different common condition. If you would like easy, practical guidance on other everyday health concerns, you may wish to explore the rest of books in this series.

Books in this series:

- Better Health starts Here: A Doctor's Guide to Staying Healthy After 40
- A Doctor's Easy Guide to Understanding & Managing OBESITY
- Doctor, What DIET Is Best for Me?
- Doctor, Why Can't I Lose Weight? A Doctor's Guide to safe & Sustainable Weight Loss)
- A Doctor's Easy Guide to GLP-1 for Obesity
- A Doctor's Easy Guide to Understanding & Managing HIGH BLOOD PRESSURE
- A Doctor's Guide to Living Well With DIABETES
- A Doctor's Guide to Understanding & Managing THYROID DISEASES
- A Doctor's Guide to Understanding & Managing HIGH CHOLESTEROL
- A Doctor's Practical Guide to HEART HEALTH After 40: How to Protect Your Heart & Live Longer
- A Doctor's Guide to Healing & Reversing FATTY LIVER DISEASE: Simple, Natural & Science-Based Steps to Reduce Liver Fat and Prevent Complications

- Control Your ACID REFLUX, HEARTBURN & GERD: A Doctor's Practical Guide that Works
- Live Comfortably with IRRITABLE BOWEL SYNDROME: A Doctor's Practical Guide to Understanding & Managing IBS
- A Doctor's Practical Guide to Understanding & Managing GALLBLADDER STONES & OTHER PROBLEMS
- Take Control of COPD: A Doctor's Practical Guide to Better Breathing
- Living Better Life with ASTHMA: A Doctor's Practical Guide to Asthma Control
- SLEEP APNEA & SNORING: A Doctor's Practical Guide to Better Sleep & Better Health
- KIDNEY STONES: A Doctor's Practical Guide to Prevention & Care
- Protect Your KIDNEYS: A Doctor's Practical Guide to Kidney Health & Prevention
- PROSTATE HEALTH After 40: A Doctor's Practical Guide to Early Detection & Care
- ARTHRITIS: A Doctor's Practical Guide to Pain Control & Mobility
- A Doctor's Practical Guide to Fixing BACK PAIN Step by Step
- A Doctor's Practical Guide to Understanding & Managing GOUT & URIC ACID and Preventing Complications
- HEALTHY SKIN & COMMON SKIN PROBLEMS: A Doctor's Practical Guide to Skin Care
- DEMENTIA & MEMORY LOSS: A Doctor's Practical Guide to Prevention & Management
- Doctor, Why Am I TIRED All The Time? Fixing Fatigue & Getting Your Energy Back

Printed by Libri Plureos GmbH in Hamburg,
Germany

9 781971 672304